This booklet explains root canal therapy:

Why it's needed,

How it's done,

And how successful it can be.

Why Root Canal Therapy? contains general principles. There are, of course, individual exceptions. Your own dentist's advice is the best advice you can get.

ANATOMY

Each tooth consists of two parts: the *crown* and the *root(s)*.

Only the crown is visible in the mouth. The roots are in the bone, under the gums.

The *gums* are a protective type of skin that clings to the necks of the teeth and covers the bone holding the teeth.

Molars are back teeth. They usually have two or three roots. Most other teeth have one root.

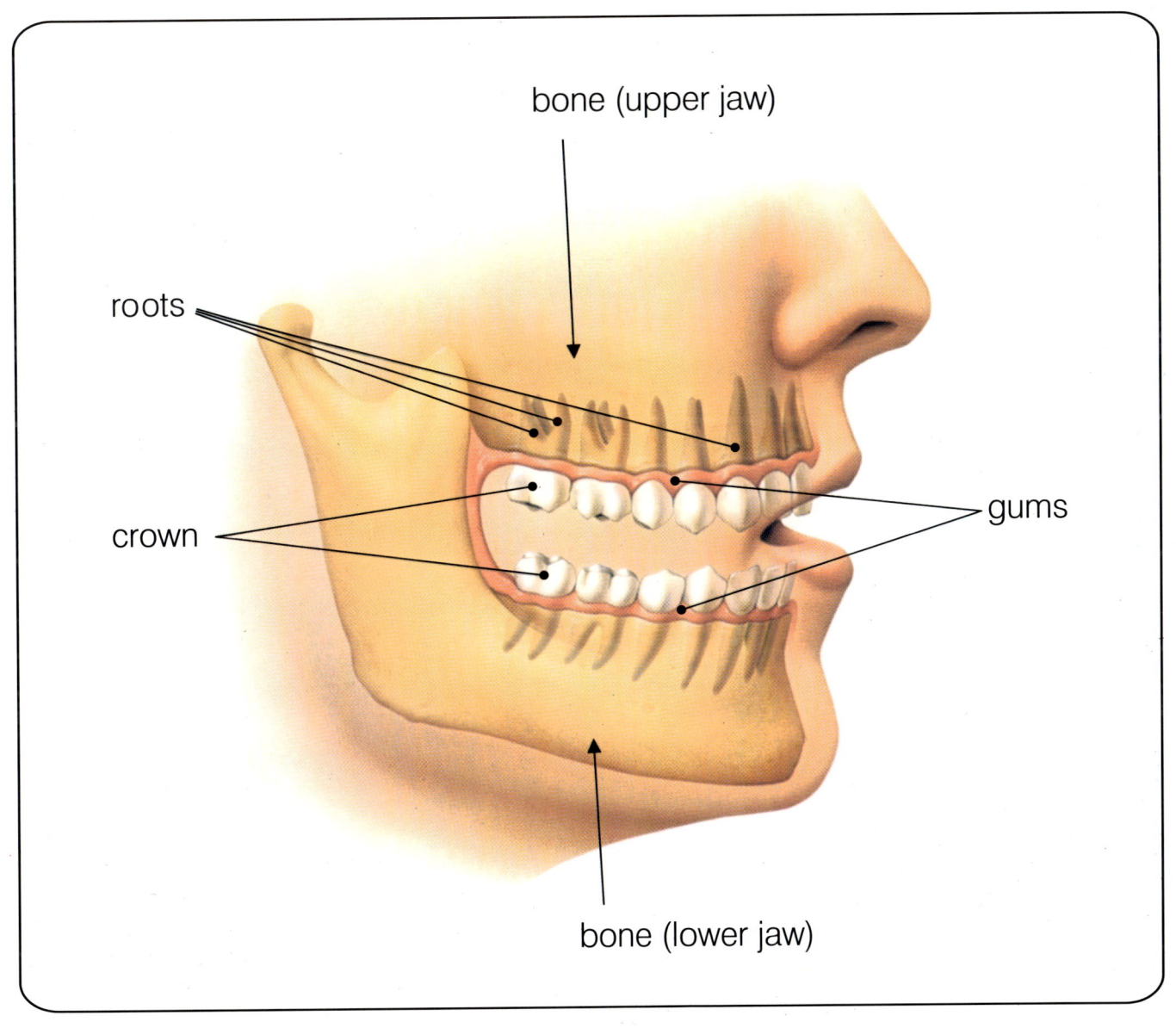

bone (upper jaw)

roots

crown

gums

bone (lower jaw)

The crown of a tooth has an outer shell made of a very hard substance called *enamel*.

The inside of the tooth is made of a less hard substance called *dentin*.

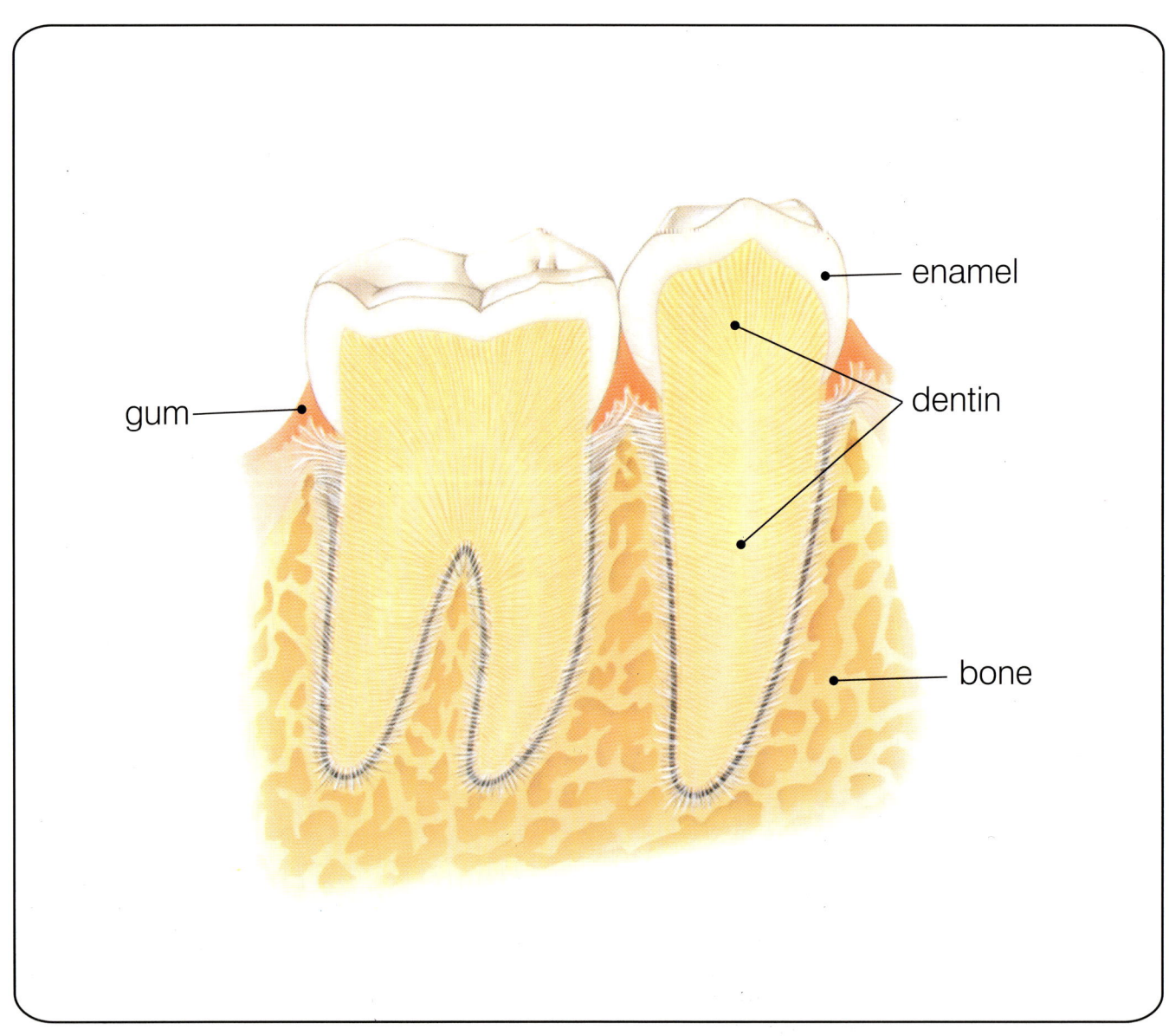

The center of the tooth is hollow.

This hollow in the crown portion of the tooth is called the *pulp chamber.*

In the root portion of the tooth, the hollow narrows to become a small canal called the *root canal.*

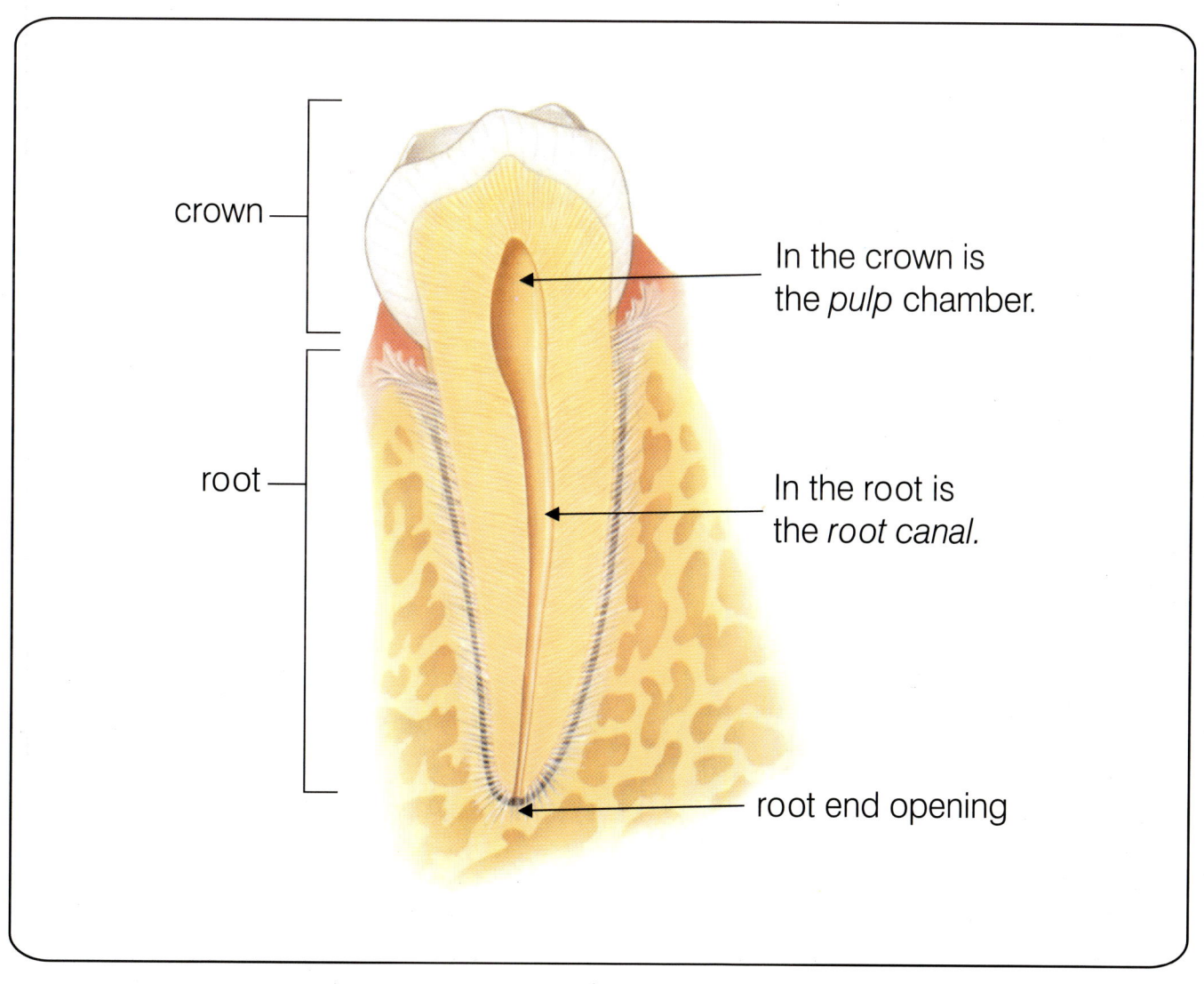

crown

root

In the crown is the *pulp* chamber.

In the root is the *root canal.*

root end opening

In teeth with more than one root, each root has its own canal that extends from the single pulp chamber.

Each root canal ends at a tiny opening at the end of the root.

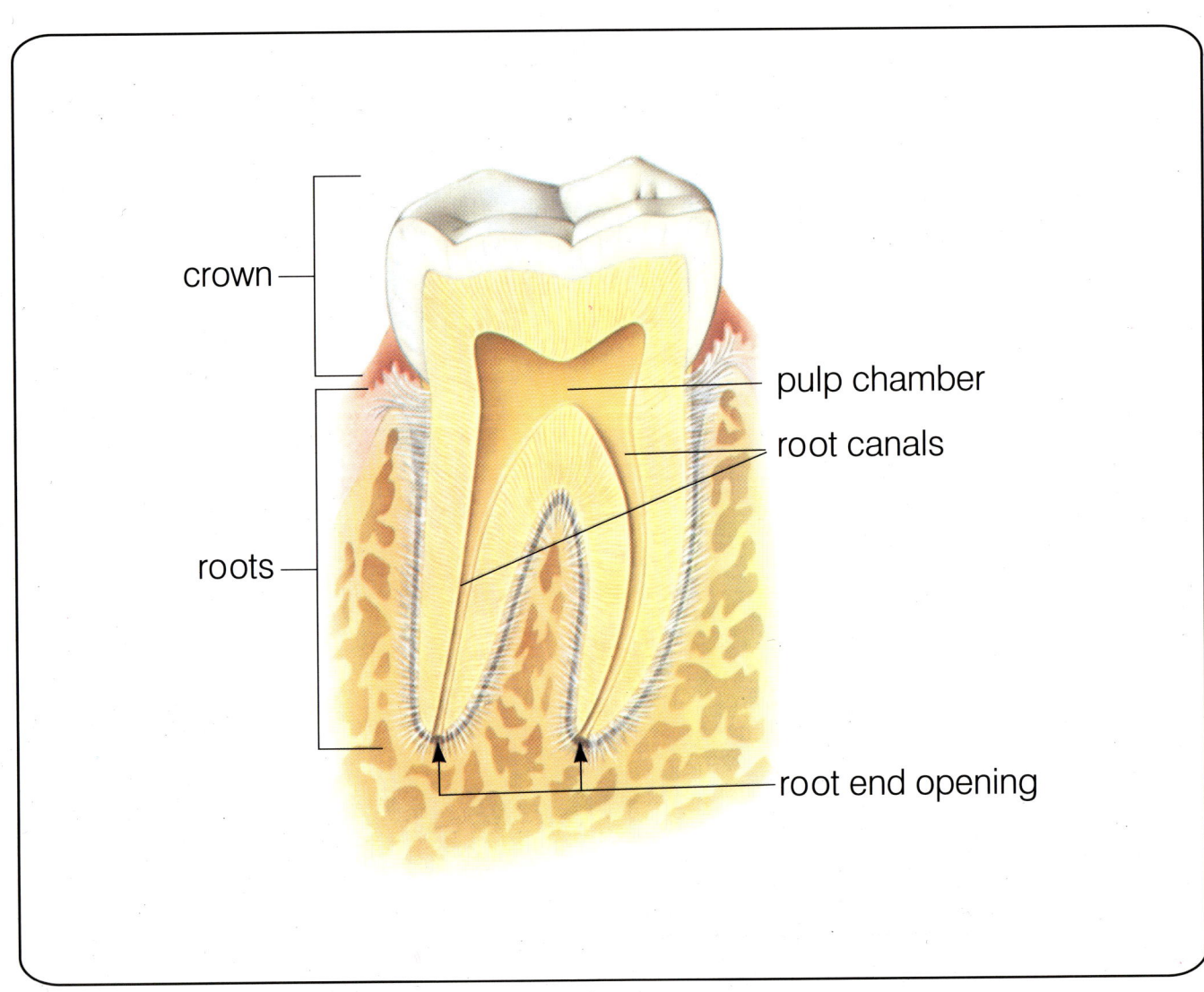

Usually there is only one canal in each root, but some teeth have more than one.

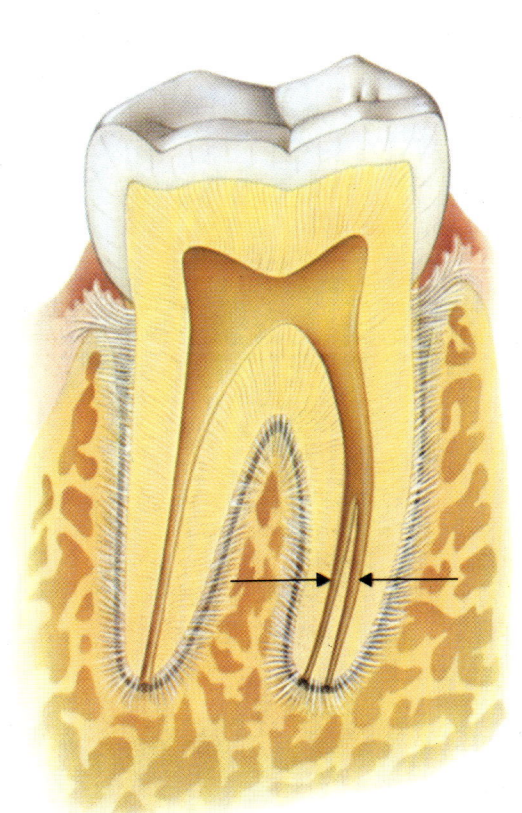

two root canal in one root

THE PULP

The pulp chamber and root canals contain a living tissue called *pulp*.

The pulp is a fine network of delicate tissue fibers. It contains small arteries, veins, and nerves that have branched off an artery, vein, and nerve that pass through the jawbone.

The arteries and veins nourish the pulp with blood. This blood supply is a source of defense against any infection of the pulp.

The pulp is often mistakenly called the nerve. But nerves are only a part of this complex living tissue.

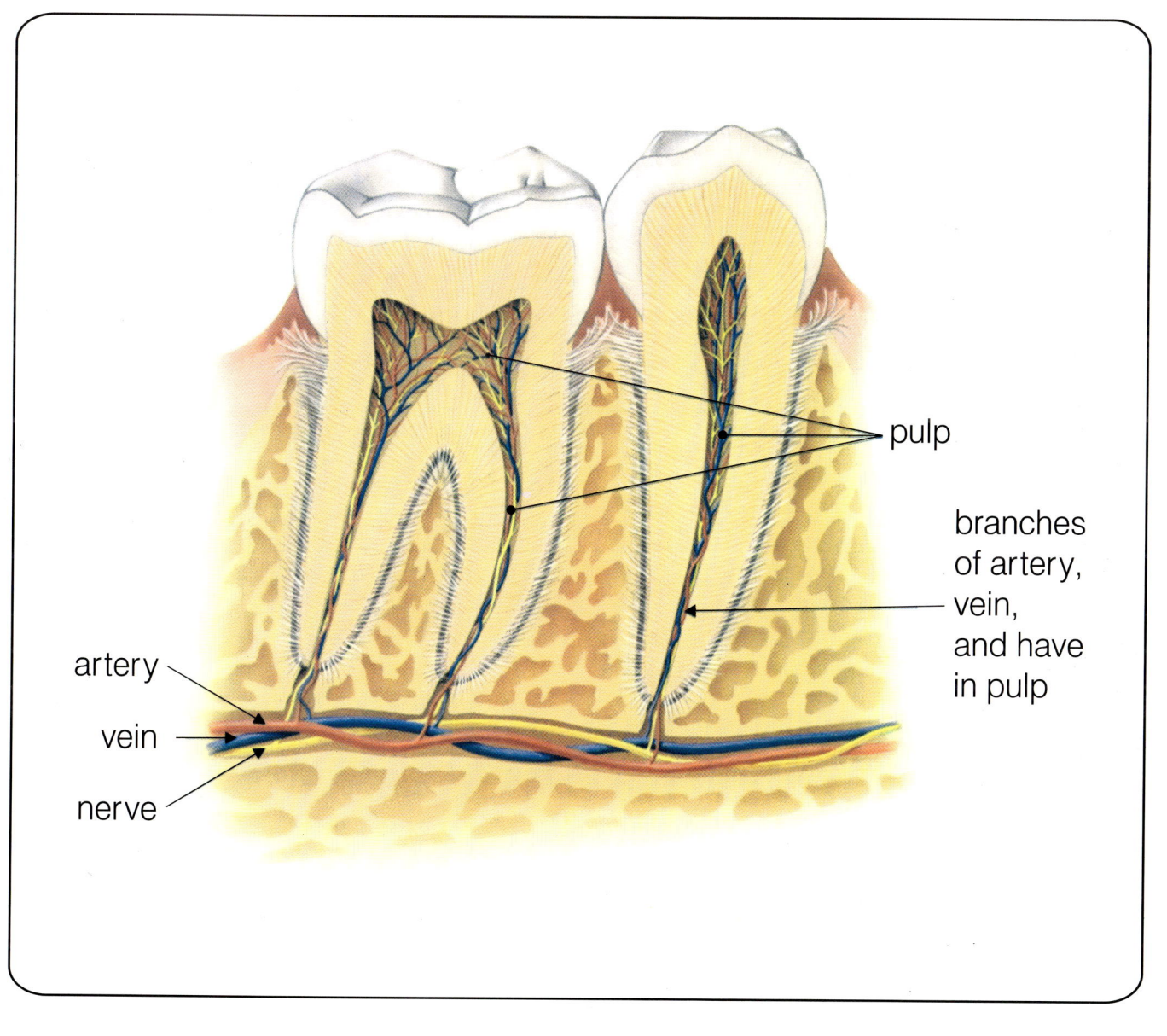

pulp

branches
of artery,
vein,
and have
in pulp

artery

vein

nerve

PULP AND JAW INFECTION

Bacteria are the most common causes of inflammation and infection of the pulp. They enter the pulp through tooth decay or if a tooth breaks.

Invading bacteria first overwhelm the pulp defenses in the pulp chamber. Then they destroy the pulp in the root canals.

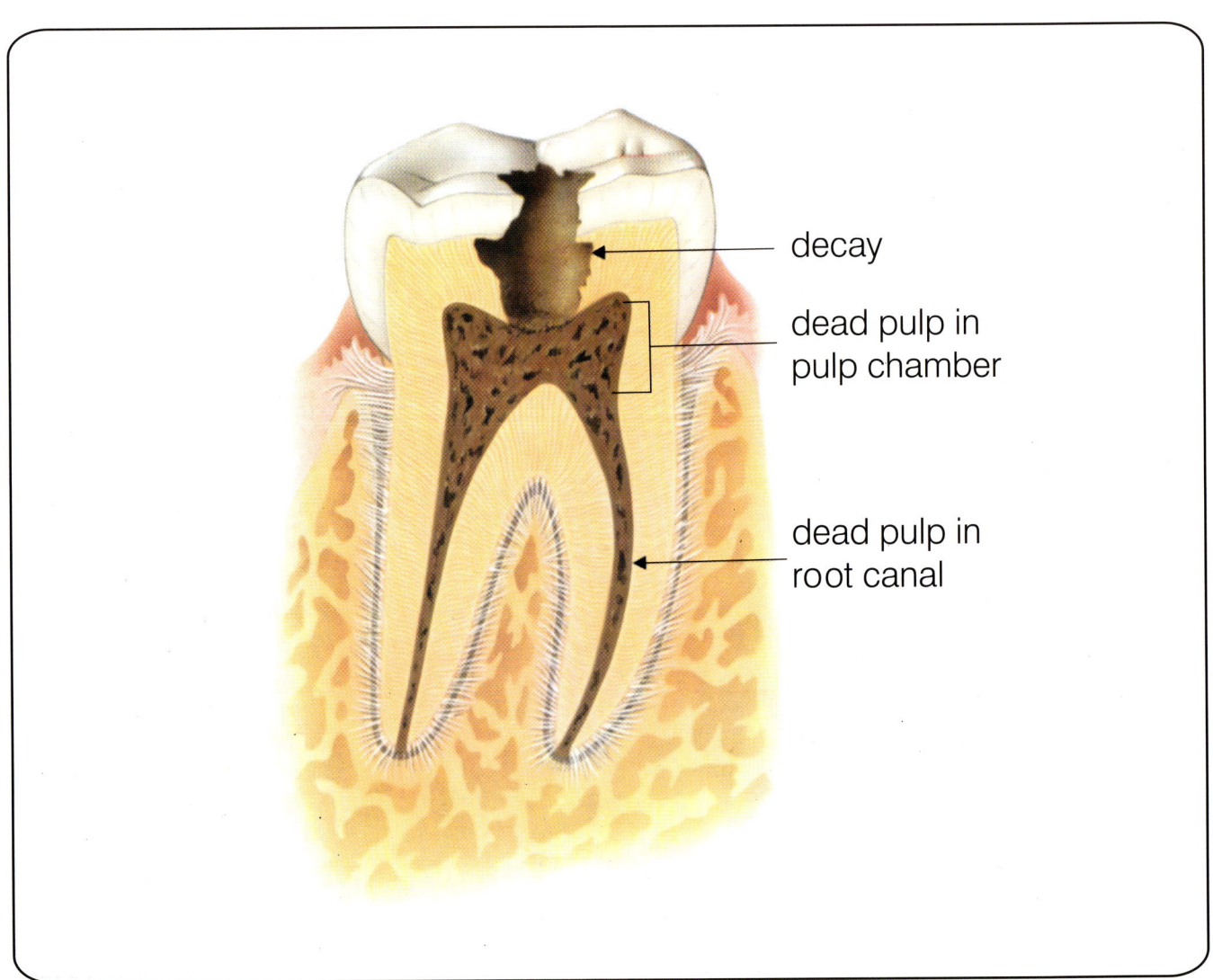

decay

dead pulp in
pulp chamber

dead pulp in
root canal

Toxins (poisons) from the bacteria that have destroyed the pulp can leak out of the root ends into the jawbone. The jawbone, like all bones, is a living tissue. It has arteries, veins, and nerves, like any other tissue. Therefore, it can become inflamed and infected by the presence of bacteria and their toxins.

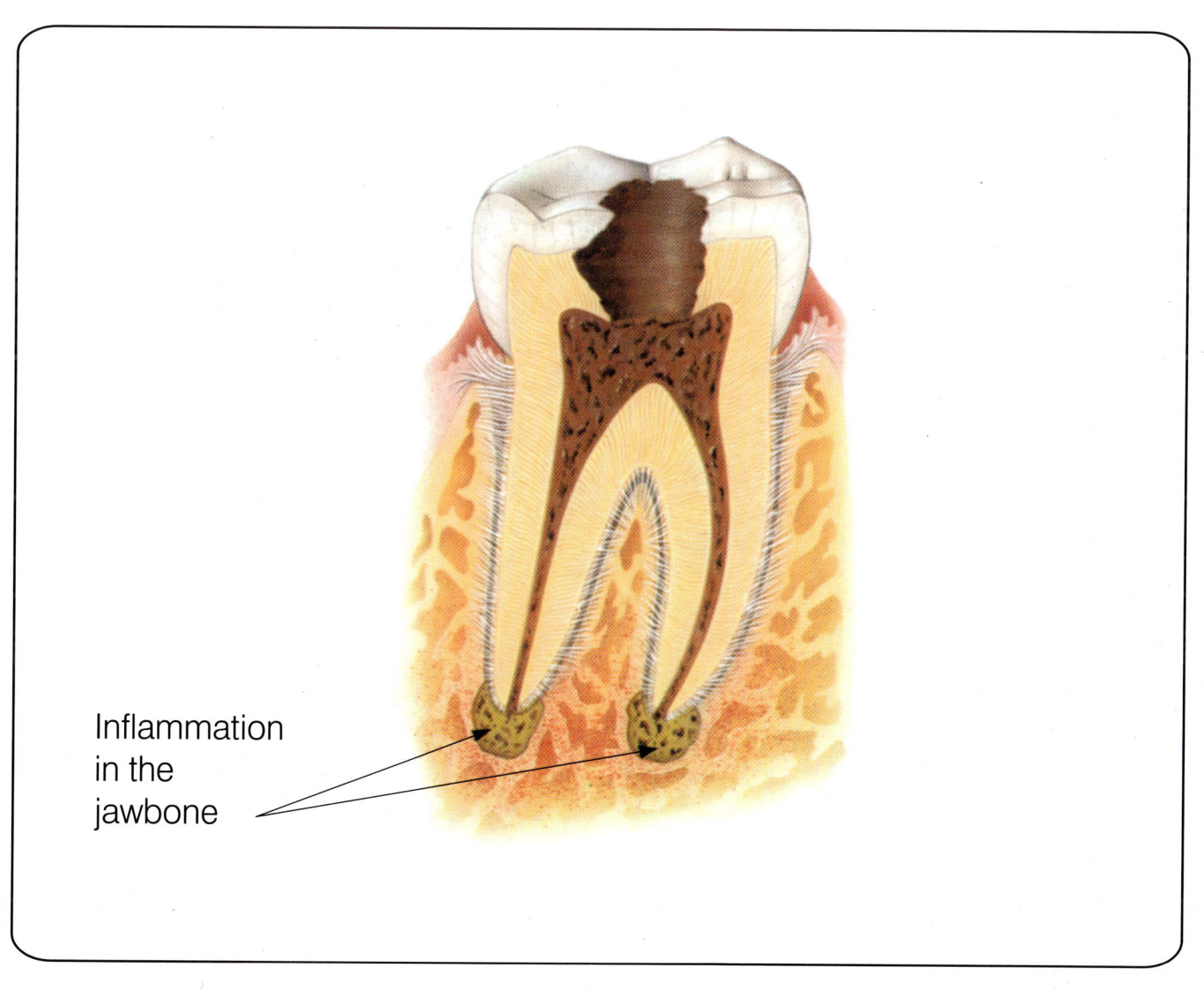

Inflammation in the jawbone

INFECTION OF THE FACE
AND NECK

Finally, long-standing dental infection in bone can erode through the side of the bone into the mouth, or into the face or neck, to cause sudden, serious, and painful swelling.

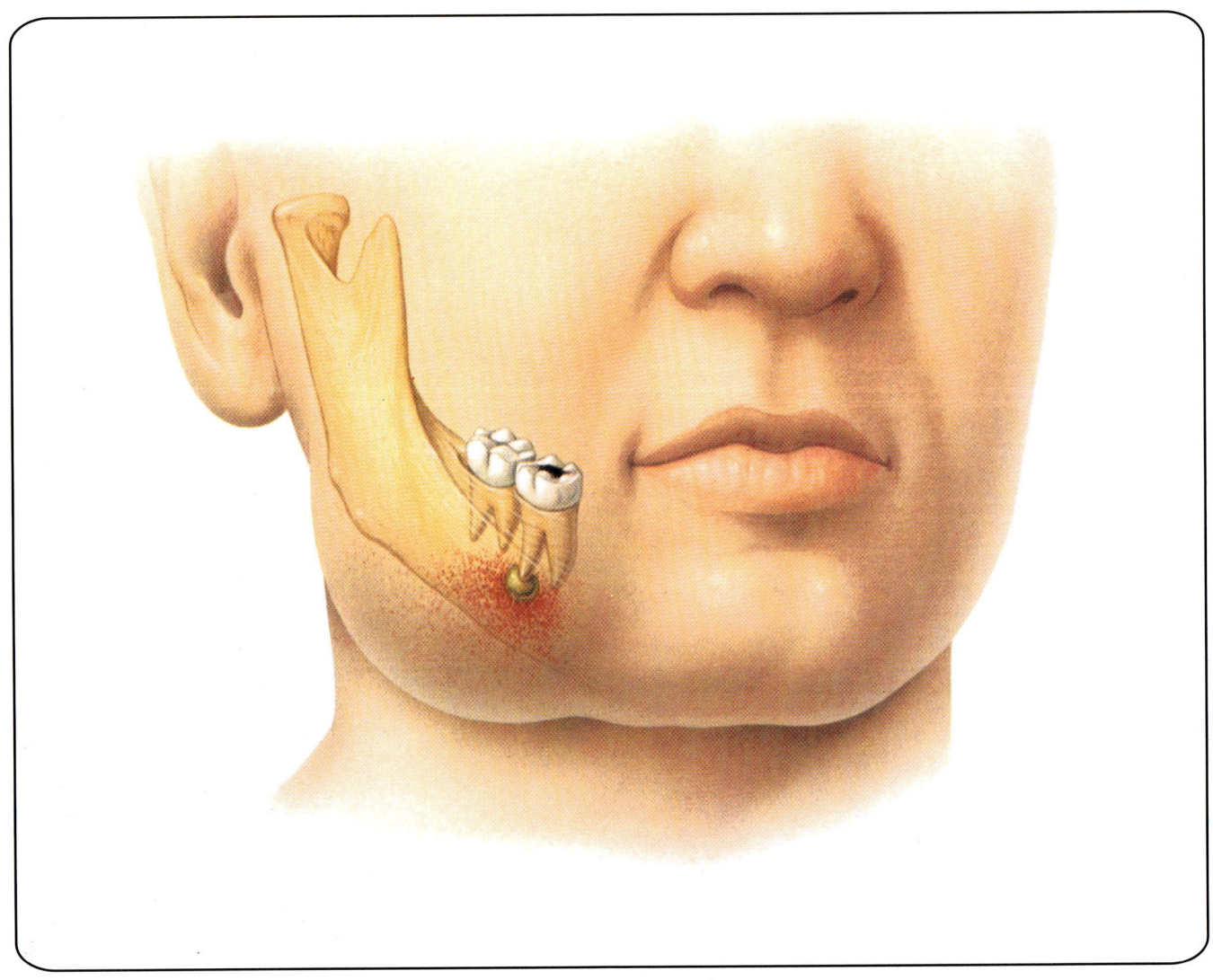

WHY ROOT CANAL THERAPY?

The goals of root canal therapy are to:

1. Remove bacteria and infected pulp from the pulp chamber and root canals.

2. Completely fill the canal(s) and pulp chamber with a solid filling material to prevent future trouble

When root canal therapy is done, inflammation in the bone around the root ends can heal, and *the tooth is saved*.

HOW ROOT CANAL THERAPY IS DONE

The method of root canal therapy shown in this booklet is a very common one. Other techniques differ in some details and materials, but accomplish the same goals.

Root canal therapy proceeds in two stages:

A. Preparing the root canal
B. Filling the canal

A. PREPARING THE ROOT CANAL

Step 1: Opening the tooth

The dentist gently makes an opening into the tooth. Local anesthesia (Novo-cain®) may be necessary to prevent pain that can occur if any nerve fibers are still alive in the pulp.

All tooth decay is removed.

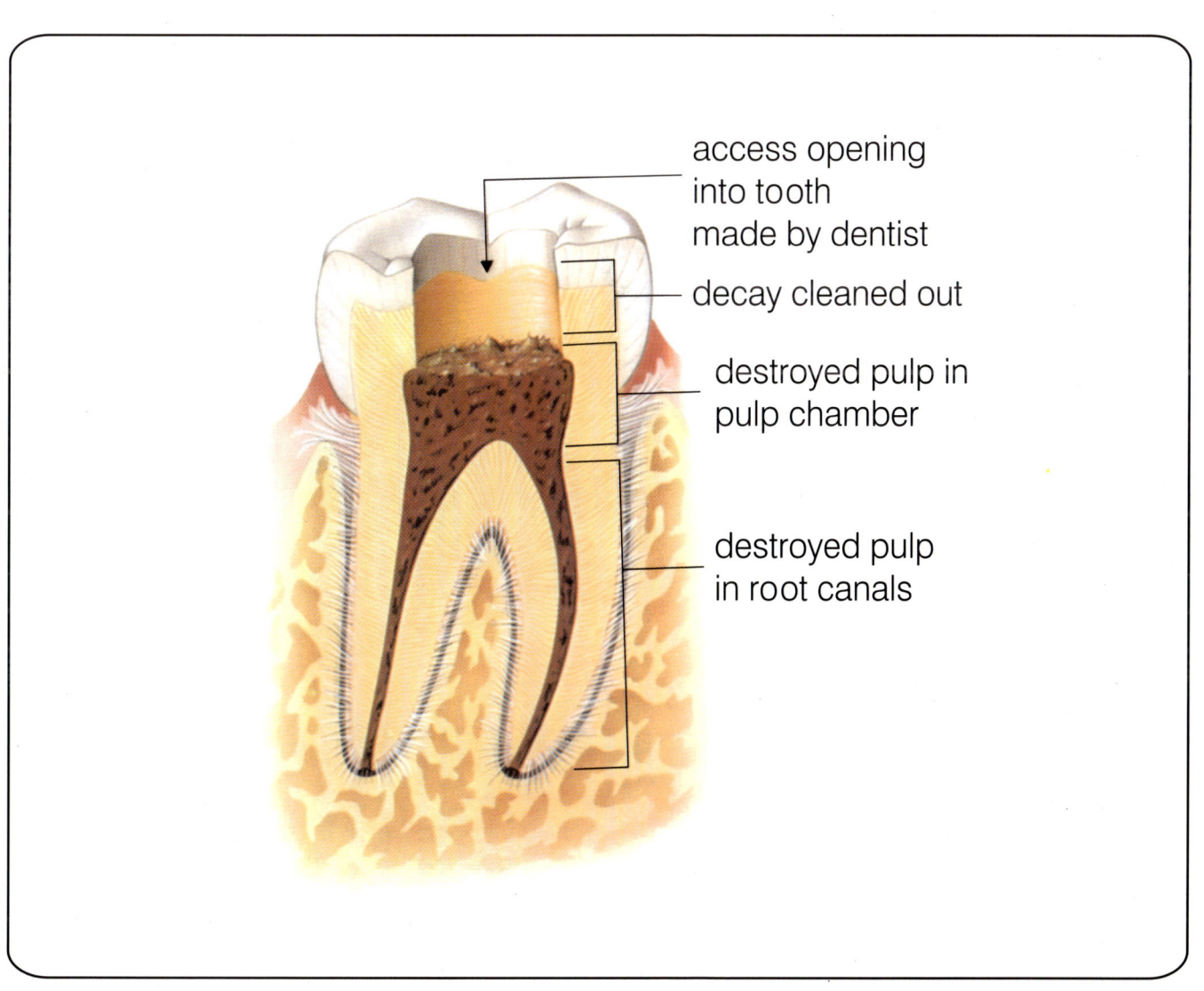

access opening
into tooth
made by dentist

decay cleaned out

destroyed pulp in
pulp chamber

destroyed pulp
in root canals

Step 2: Shaping the canals

The dentist uses a series of very delicate, flexible finger-held instruments. The one used in the illustration is a *file*.

Each file the dentist uses is slightly larger than the preceding one. The canals are delicately cleaned with these instruments to remove dead pulp debris and bacteria.

The dentist then shapes each canal to receive a filling.

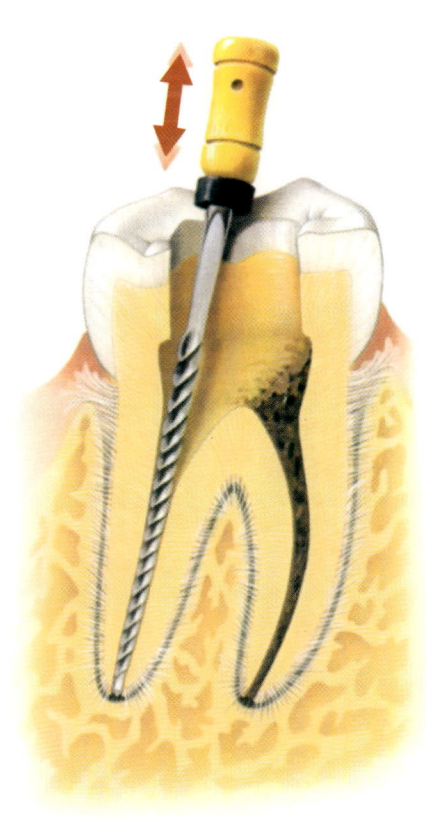

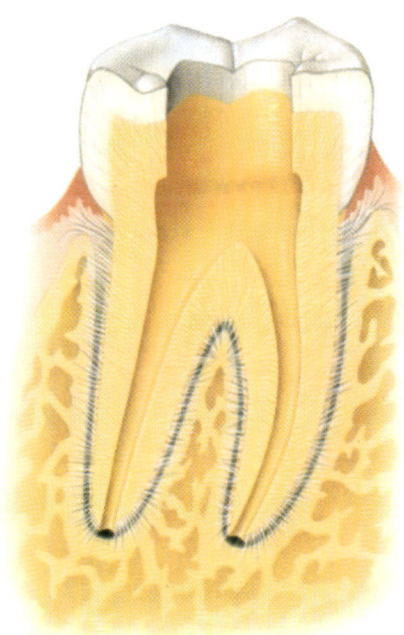

A file is used to clean and then shape the canals.

The canals are now prepared (shaped) to receive the root canal filling.

X-rays help assure that the instruments go exactly to the end of the root and not beyond.

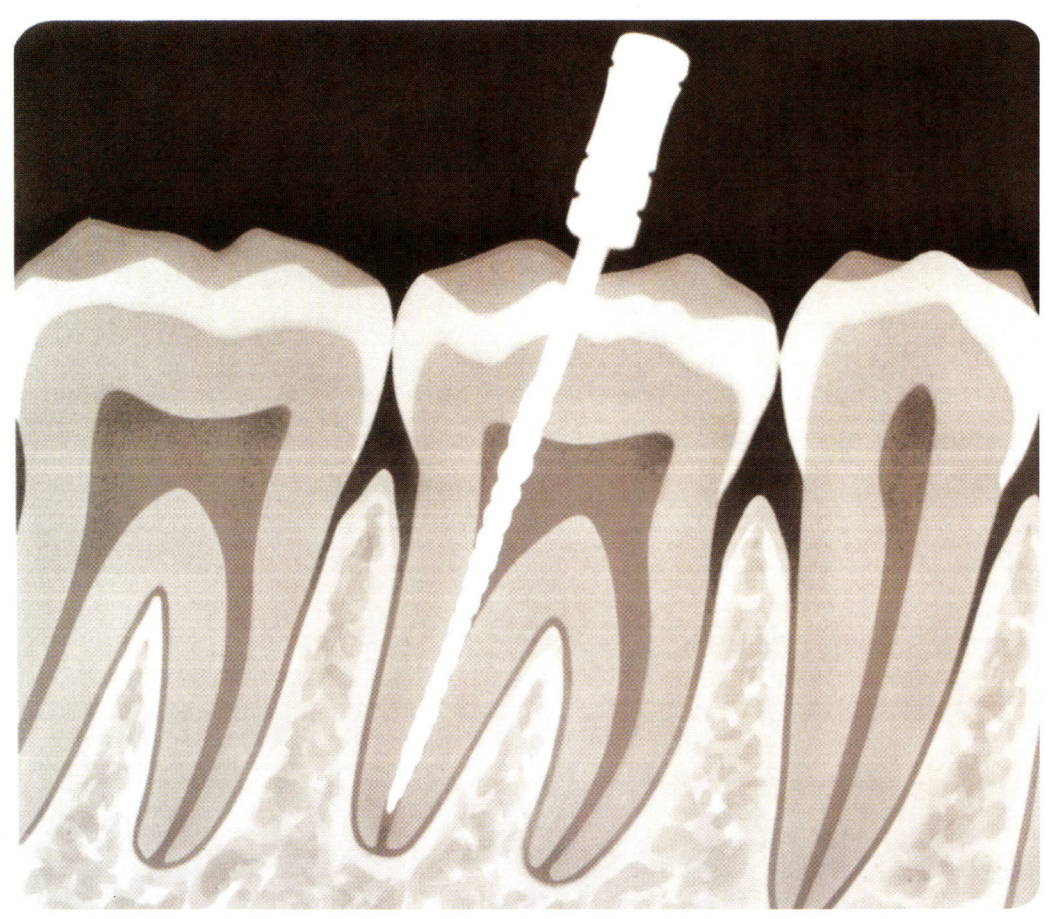

X-ray showing the file is not yet to the end of the root.

Canal preparation may take several visits, especially for difficult curved or narrow canals.

After preparation, *all canals must be solidly filled*. Otherwise, tissue fluid from the bone could eventually seep into any unfilled areas of the canal, decaying there into toxic products. These toxic products will then seep out of the root end into the bone to cause more inflammation.

B. FILLING THE CANALS

The most commonly used filling material is a firm, waxy, rubbery compound called *gutta-percha*. It is manufactured into long, thin, tapering cones called gutta-percha *points*.

Step 1

The first gutta-percha point is inserted into the prepared canal. It matches the size of the last and largest file used.

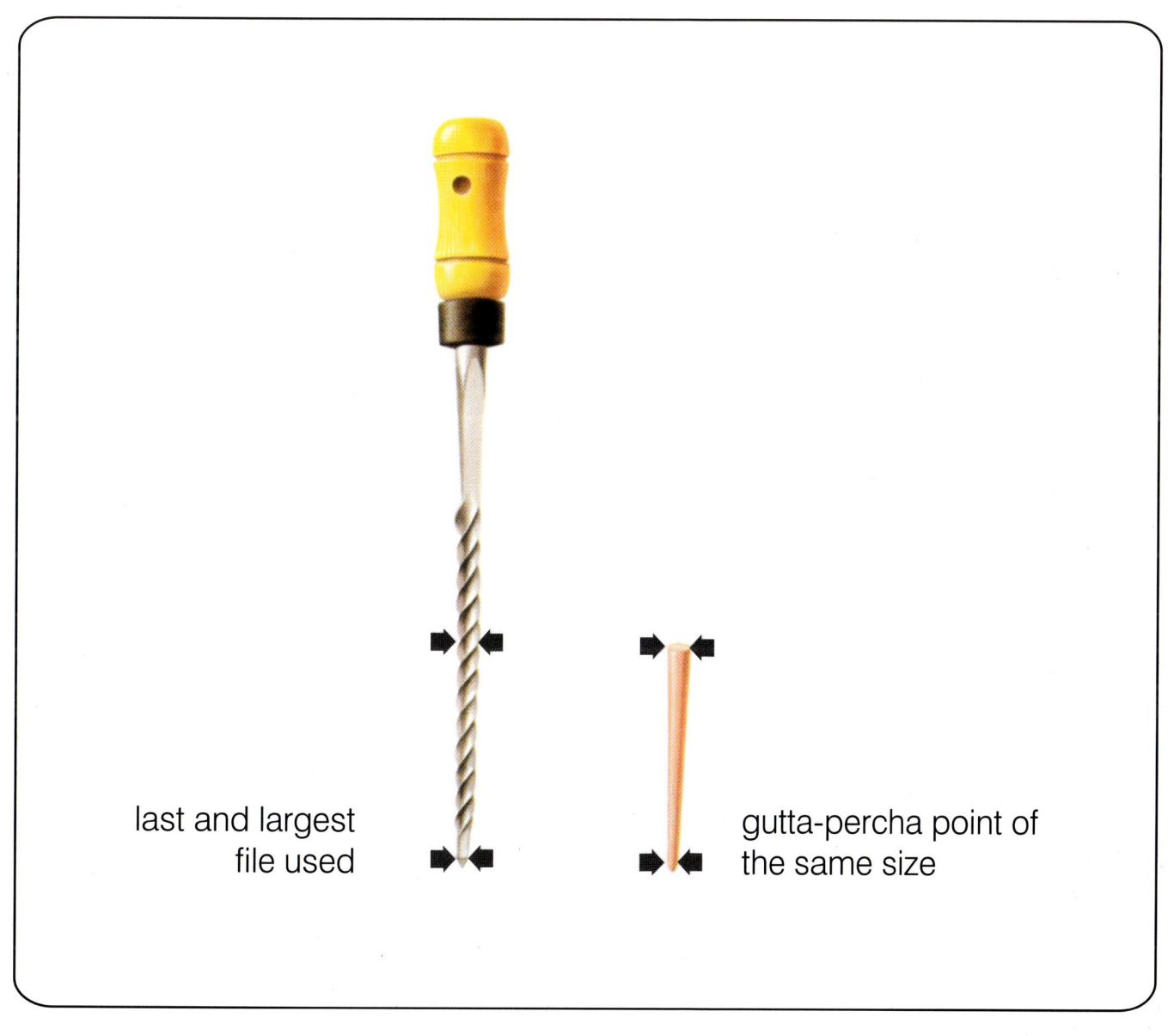

last and largest file used

gutta-percha point of the same size

Step 2

The dentist coats this point with a special liquid cement. The coated point is then inserted firmly to the end of the root. Wedged tightly, it *completely seals off the end of the canal* so that no fluids can leak past it.

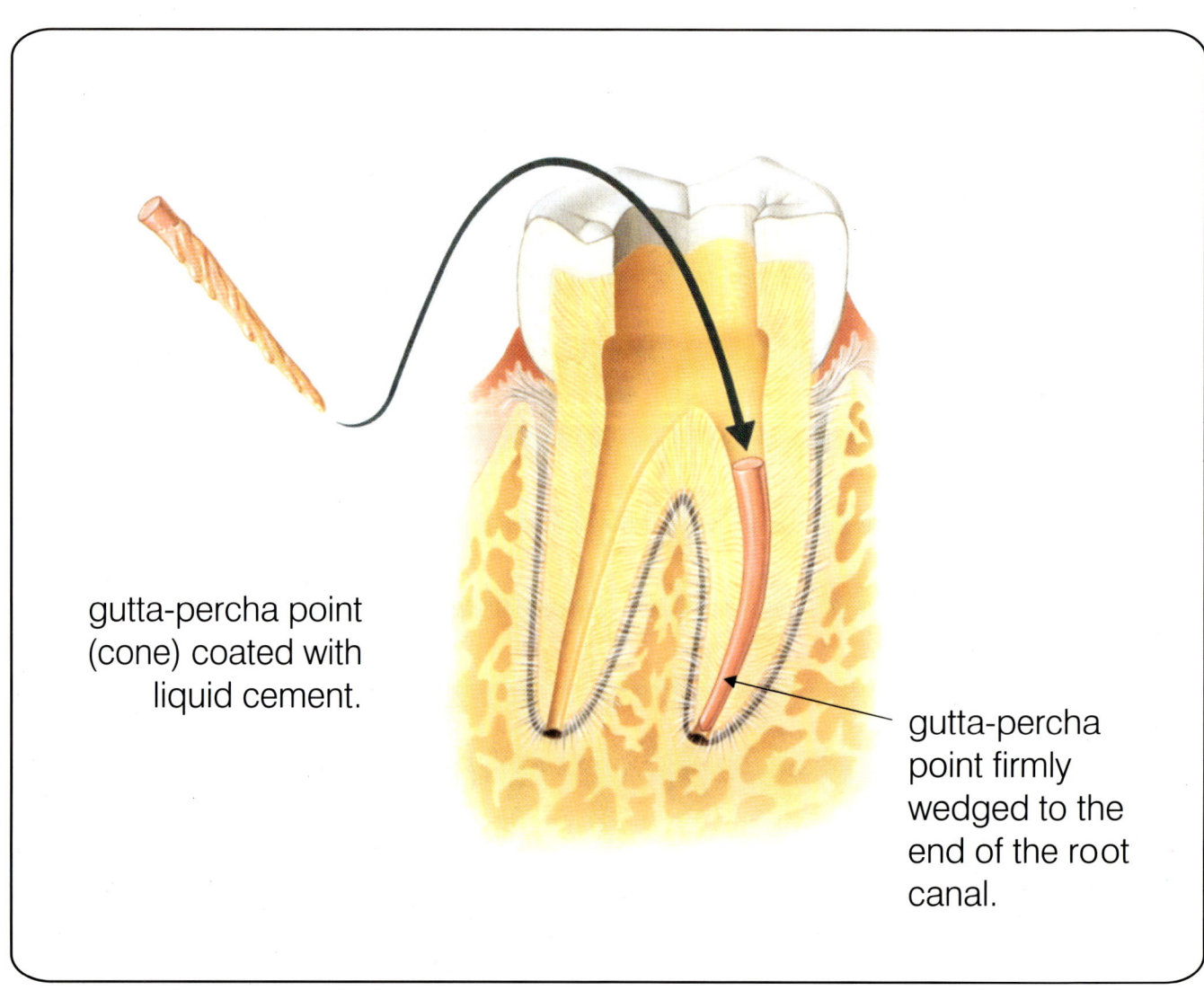

gutta-percha point (cone) coated with liquid cement.

gutta-percha point firmly wedged to the end of the root canal.

Step 3

The dentist now packs the remaining portion of each canal with gutta–percha pieces up to the level of the pulp chamber.

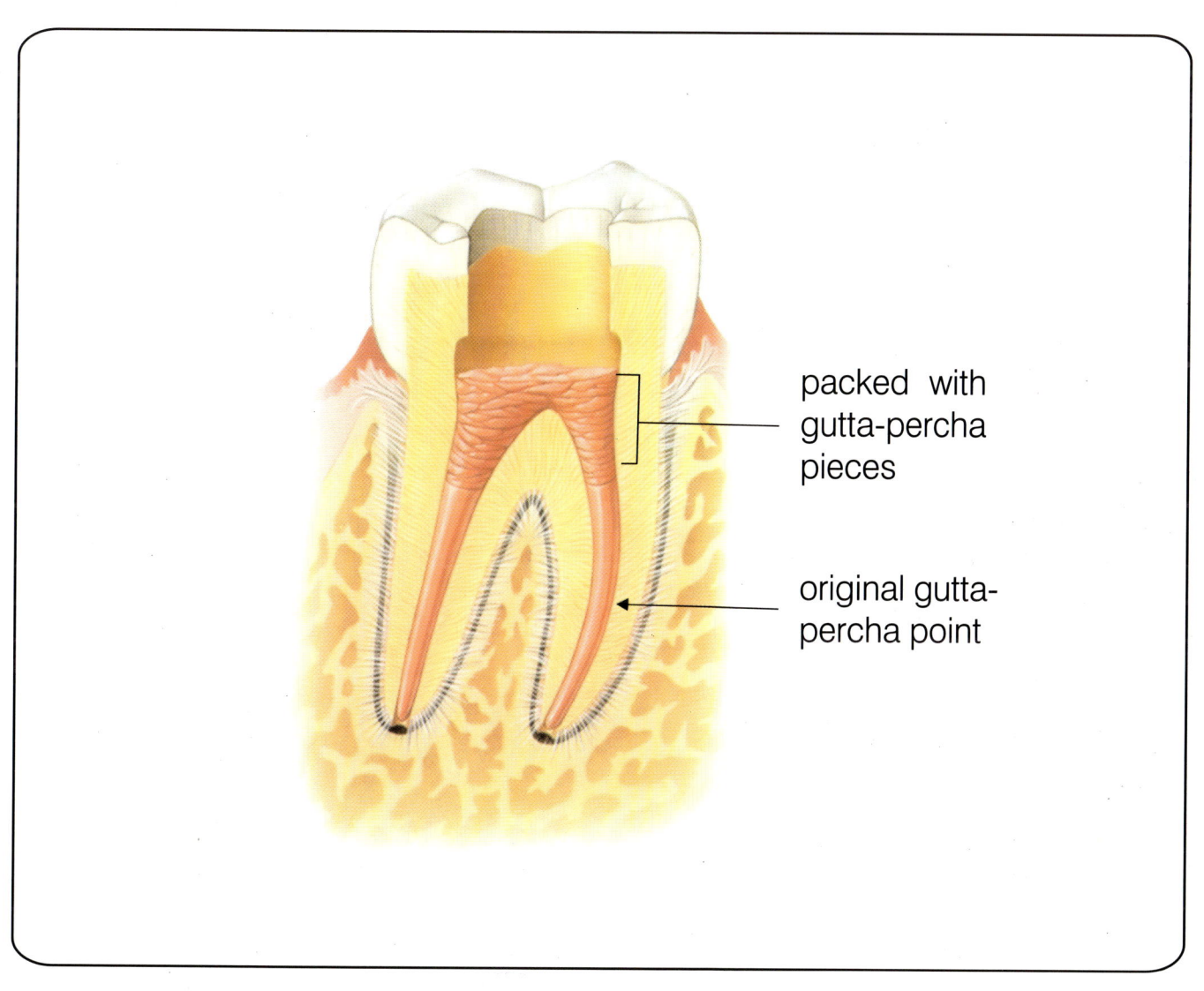

packed with gutta-percha pieces

original gutta-percha point

Step 4

Lastly, the dentist fills the tooth with a temporary protective cement.

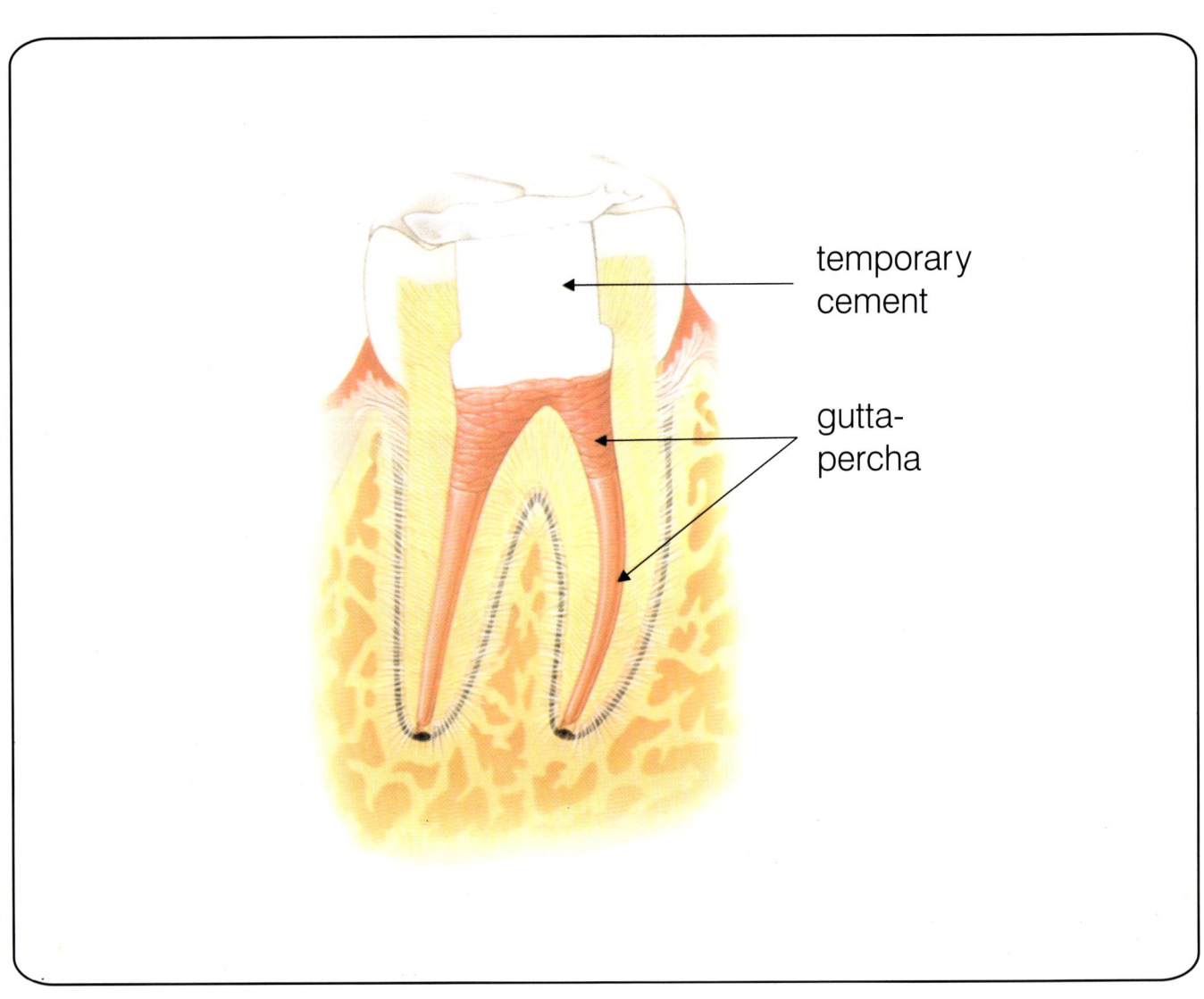

temporary
cement

gutta-
percha

RESTORING THE TOOTH AFTER ROOT CANAL THERAPY

Now that root canal therapy is finished, the dentist can repair the brokendown tooth crown that was damaged by decay.

Tooth decay that was bad enough to let bacteria into the pulp usually has destroyed much of the crown. Cleaning and shaping the canals further weakens the tooth. Such a tooth may break during chewing unless repair includes an internal *post* support followed by a fully covering crown.

PLACING POSTS

There are many internal post placement methods, all requiring great care and precision. One approach for a badly broken-down lower molar is illustrated on the following two pages.

Placing Post in a Badly Broken-Down Lower Molar

Root canal therapy is completed.

The temporary filling is taken out, and two-thirds of the gutta-percha is removed from the left root. A stainless steel post is inserted.

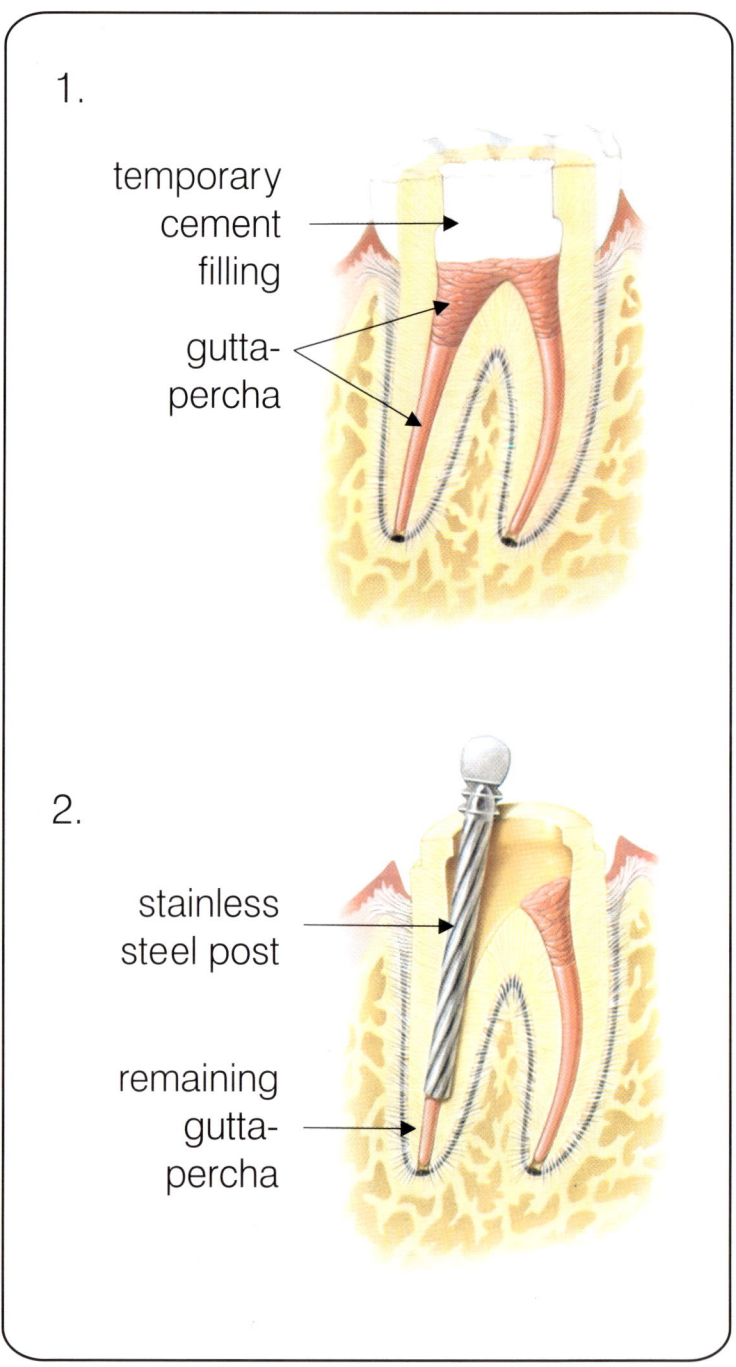

1. temporary cement filling
   gutta-percha

2. stainless steel post
   remaining gutta-percha

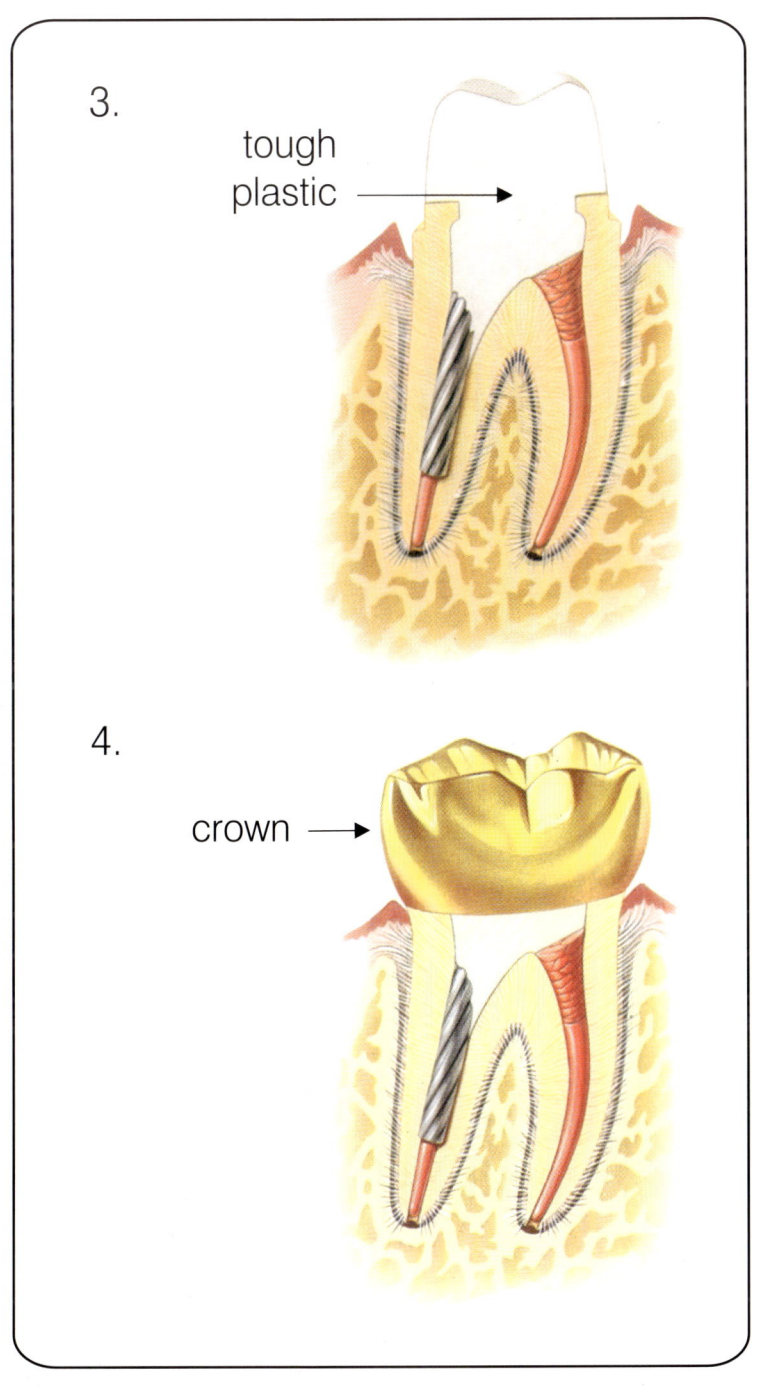

3.

tough plastic →

4.

crown →

A plastic mix flows into the tooth and around the post, and is built up well above the gum. It hardens and then is shaped to receive a crown.

A crown is precision-fitted.

COMMON QUESTIONS AND THEIR ANSWERS

Q. Is root canal therapy painful?

A. Local anesthesia (Novocain®) can make most teeth painless to treat.

Between treatments, aspirin-strength medications usually work well. Occasionally, dentist must write a prescription for a stronger pain reliever.

Q. Isn't root canal therapy quite expensive?

A. It's not, considering the time, patience, and skill needed to perform it. And the cost of root canal therapy is substantially less than the cost of a bridge needed to replace a tooth lost because root canal therapy was *not* done.

Q. What is an endodontist?

A. An endodontist is a root canal therapy specialist. After four years of dental school, he or she takes two years of intensive specialty training. An endodontist does both routine and complicated root canal cases.

Q. Despite a dentist's or endodontist's best effort, don't some root canal therapies fail?

A. Seldom. The odds for success in uncomplicated cases are excellent; in fact, they are *well over 90%*.

Q. Why do the rare failures happen?

A. Usually due to special complications. Illustrations of some of these complications follow.

Accessory Root Canals

Some teeth have large side canals coming off the main canal, most often near the root end. These cannot be cleaned out, and the bacteria they contain may keep a root-end inflammation going after the main canal is filled.

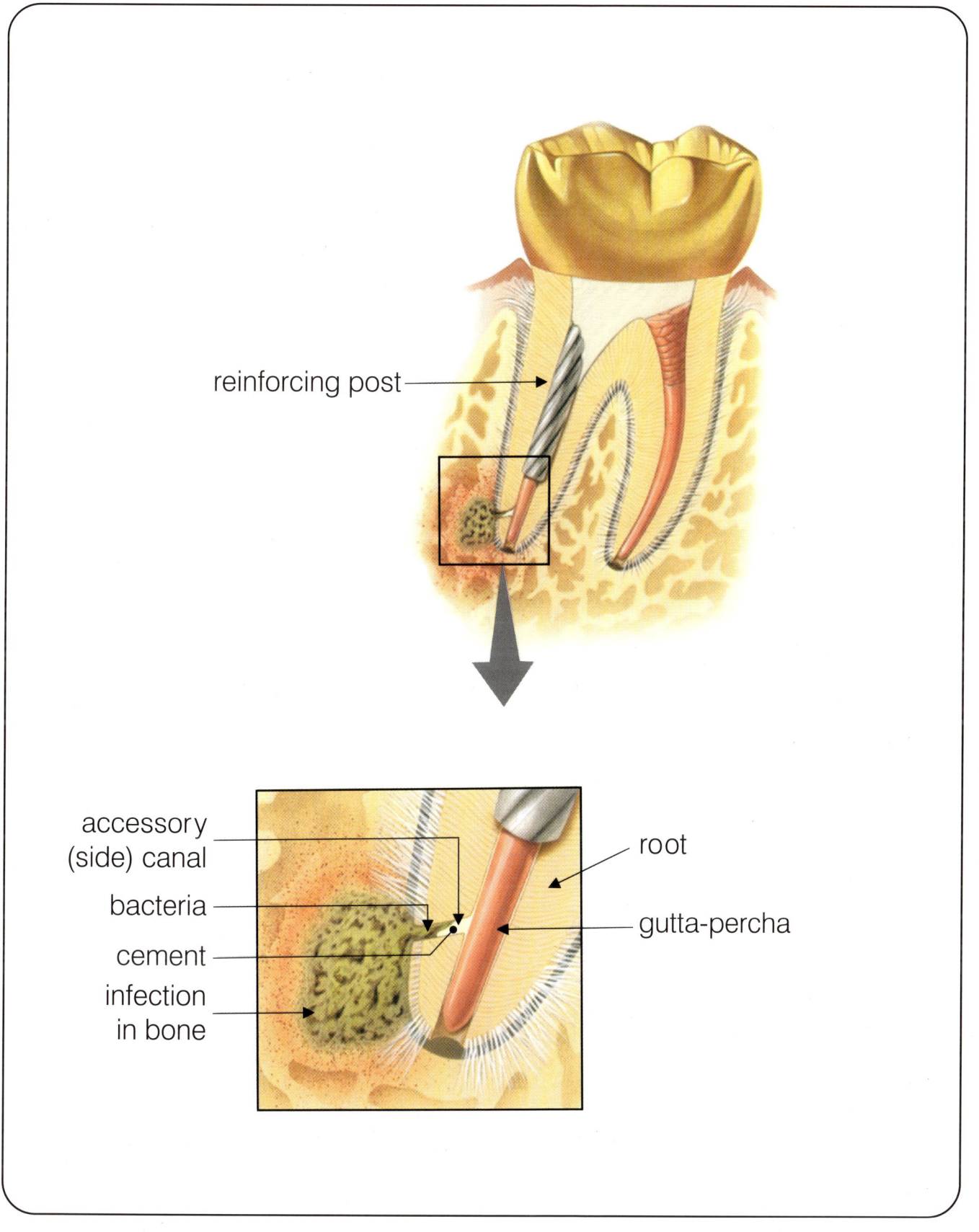

reinforcing post

accessory
(side) canal

bacteria

cement

infection
in bone

root

gutta-percha

Badly Curved Roots

It is not possible to treat severely curved root canals. Bacteria still left in the ends of these roots can continue to infect the surrounding bone after root canal therapy.

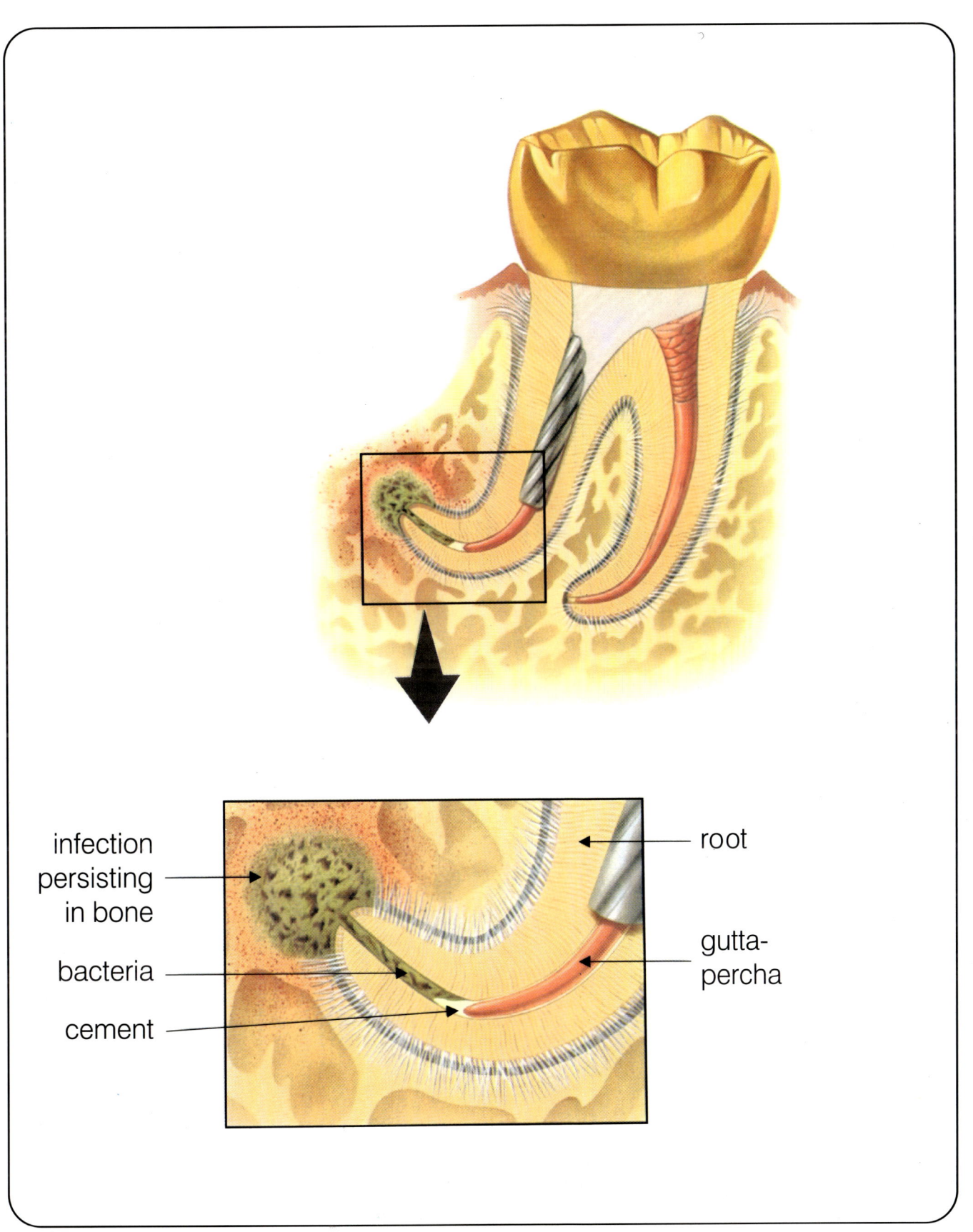

infection persisting in bone

bacteria

cement

root

gutta-percha

Very Narrow Canals

Some canals become exceedingly narrow, especially in the teeth of older people, or in teeth with deep fillings.

It was impossible to prepare the tiny lower ends of the canals of this tooth. These canals, each only the width of a hair, contain bacteria that can cause continuing trouble.

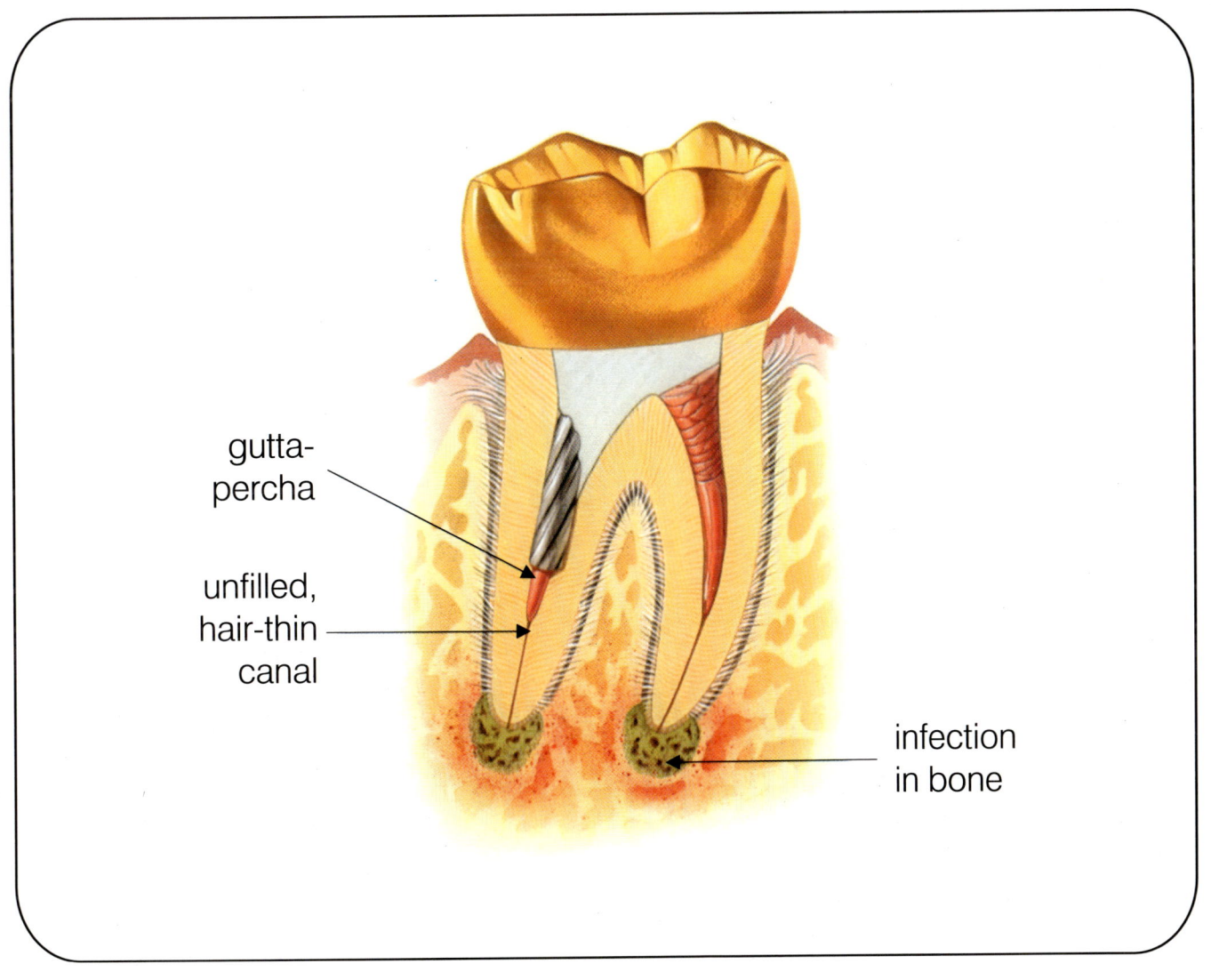

gutta-
percha

unfilled,
hair-thin
canal

infection
in bone

Cracked Root

A tooth can develop a hairline crack in its root, a crack so small i*t won't show on an X-ray*, but still large enough to harbor bacteria that can do damage.

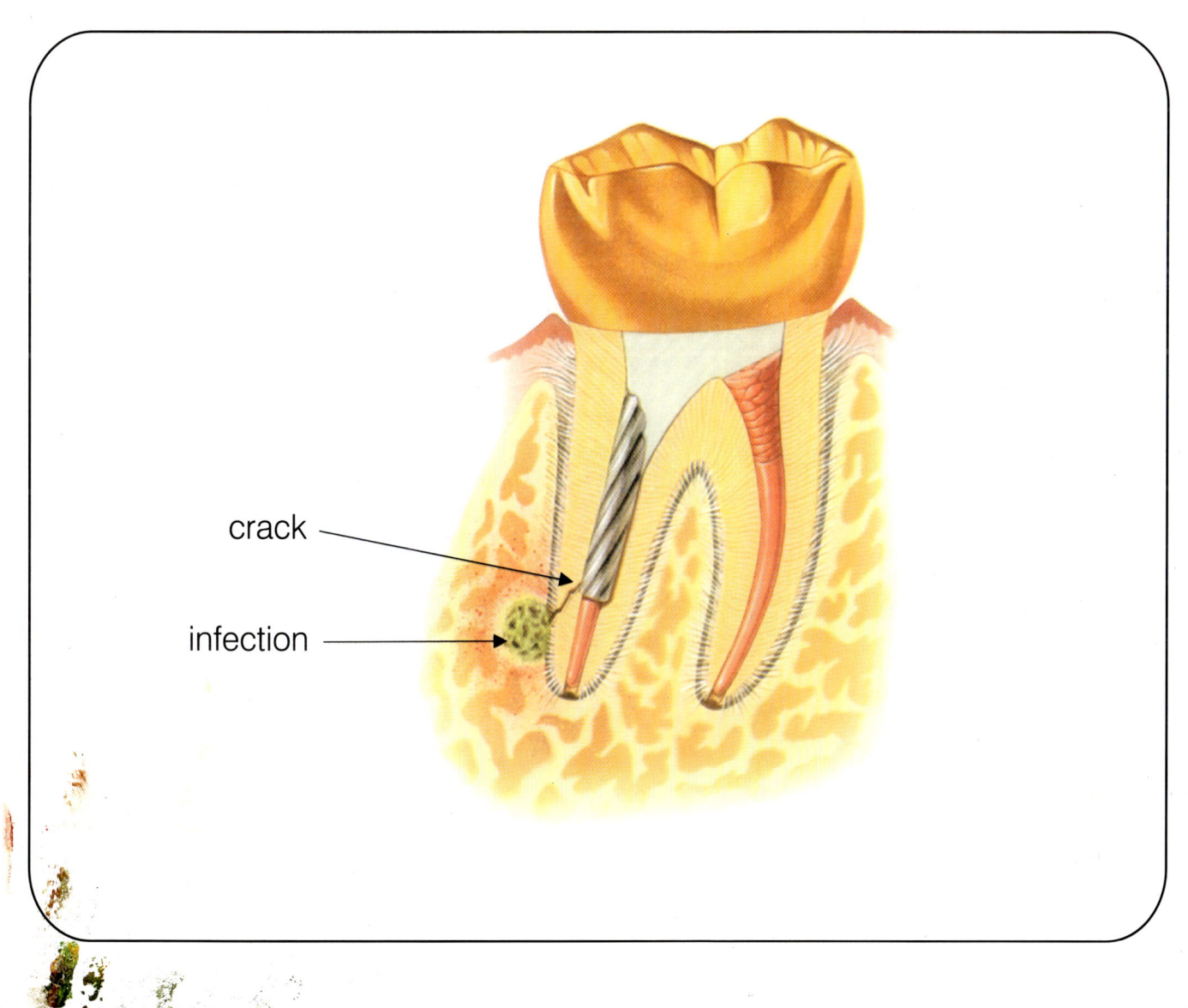

crack

infection

Q. Does failed root canal therapy mean the tooth must be extracted (taken out)?

A. Usually not. There are special techniques of canal retreatment. And, when a good seal at the end of a root is impossible to attain, the root end can frequently be surgically removed to solve the problem.

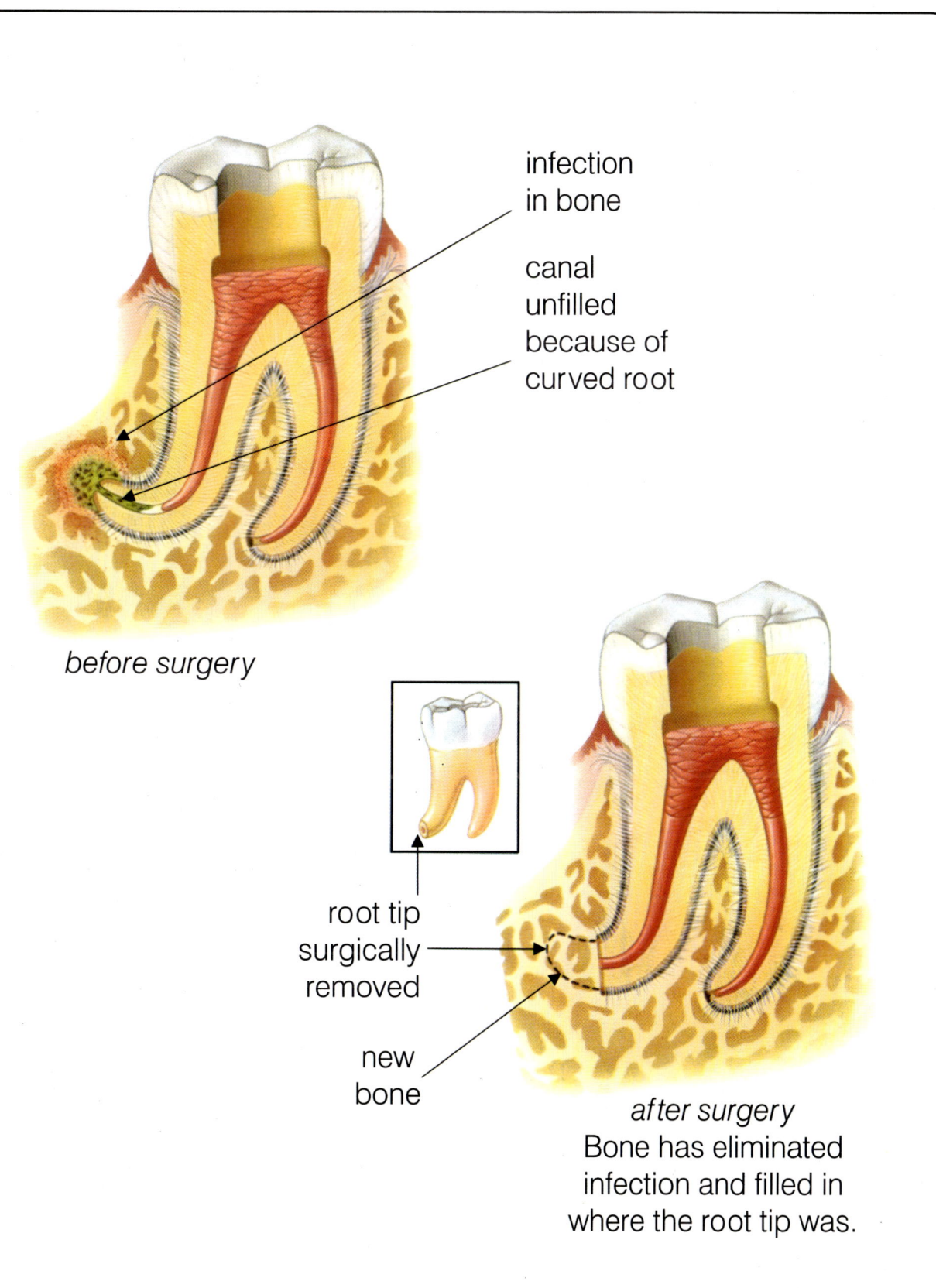

infection
in bone

canal
unfilled
because of
curved root

before surgery

root tip
surgically
removed

new
bone

after surgery
Bone has eliminated
infection and filled in
where the root tip was.

CONCLUSION

Root canal therapy saves teeth with infected pulps. It avoids the complication and greater expense of replacing teeth that would otherwise be lost.